Planning Nutritious Meals in 4 Easy Steps

Tools, Ideas, and Recipes to Make Healthy Eating Less Stressful

---

Other works by Andrea Flowers Groon, Nutrition Andrea

Available from NutritionAndrea.com or Lulu.com

- The Meal Plan for Life: Easy Clean Nutrition That's Sustainable

- Nutrition Andrea Cooks

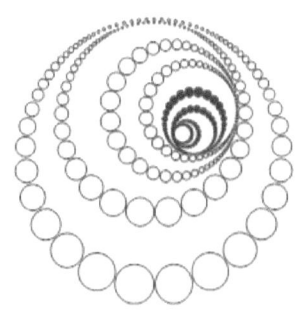

Nutrition Andrea

Planning Nutritious Meals in 4 Easy Steps

Tools, Ideas, and Recipes to Make Healthy Eating Less Stressful

Andrea@NutritionAndrea.com
http://www.NutritionAndrea.com
Twitter @NutritionAndrea
Instagram Nutrition_Andrea
Facebook.com/NutritionAndrea

Contents

Introduction

How do I get a healthy dinner on the table in 30 minutes or less after a long day at work?

I get this question from clients each week: They want to eat at home more often, provide healthy meals for their families, and get food on the table fast. Based on what they tell me, one of the biggest things preventing my clients from achieving a healthy family dinner is having "at-the-ready" menu ideas and quick recipes. Another major challenge is the time it takes to prepare, cook, and then eat by a reasonable hour. This guide will help you to organize meal planning and prepare healthy meals using just a few steps and ingredients.

I have struggled with managing a busy schedule and meal preparation over the years so I understand the problem. I am a busy, single working mom with active kids and a business to run. I have used these tools, modified them over the years and decreased my stress levels. In this guide, I will provide you with meal planning tools that are practical, sustainable, and easy to use. I now manage to cook homemade meals, most of the time, using the tools I am going to share!

How do you know if this guide is for you?

- Your goal is to eat at home more often.

- You want to prepare and eat foods that nourish the body.
- You want meal preparation to be less stressful.
- You have basic cooking skills in place.
- You are looking for a structured method of meal planning.
- You are prepared with basic cooking tools.

Step One: Plan the Menu

One of the most commonly asked questions among family members is, "What's for dinner?" And this is usually asked an hour or so before dinnertime, when people start to get hungry. Or you get the text – what are we having for dinner? By planning ahead, we can lessen the impulse to grab a fast but unhealthy dinner on the way home.

Using the resources in this book, you will have a reference list of ideas and menu plans that are nutritious, quick, and easy to prepare. The next time you are asked, "What's for dinner?" you will have a plan and an answer! Ideally, you will be able to have a plan for the week, a grocery list, and lots of options from which to choose.

A. What Does Your Family Eat?
The first step is to figure out what your family likes to eat.
- What do you eat on a regular basis?
- Are there foods that are consistently requested or your go-to quick & easy meal?
- Does anyone have a food allergy?
- Are there picky eaters you have to work around?

The nutrition guidelines recommend limiting red meat to no more than once per week, including pork.

Most families eat slightly differently on the Spring/Summer [light and fresh] than they do in the Fall/Winter [heartier and hot meals]. Consider this as you create a list.

B. Create the Menu Plan

There are several methods to create a menu plan. Use the Weekly Menu Planner [included in this book] to write the weeks' menu and necessary ingredients.

Mix and Match Method

This method uses the Mix and Match List found in the appendix.

- Select one item from each column
- Write it on the Weekly Menu Planner (included in this book)
- Write the ingredients needed and add to grocery list.

This method does not include casseroles or combination dishes but you can combine items to create one. It also provides ideas and direction for those that need some ideas or increased variety.

Suggested Menu Plans

I have provided two weeks of Sample Menu Plans and Recipes in the Appendix.

There are also ideas for using a rotisserie chicken in multiple ways, suggested salad combinations, and easy recipes. Use these ideas to add to your standard menu items or just for a change of pace!

C. Grocery List

Each family should have a Master Grocery List. This will list items you need each week – breakfast items, snacks for home and office, lunch box items, paper products, etc. Print several copies and then each week add the necessary items to the list, based on the Weekly Menu Planner. Keep the list in a prominent place so items can be added as you run out.

With any method you choose to use:

- Write the chosen foods/menu items on the Weekly Menu Planner (included in this book).
- Add the necessary ingredients to your master grocery list.
- If items repeat, like onions or chicken, determine the total amount needed for the week.
- Take stock of the items you already have on hand and adjust the amount needed accordingly.

You are now set for a week of healthy meals!

Step Two: Get the Food in the House

You have the menu planned and the grocery list is ready. Great Job!

Even with the best of intentions and plans, the practical issue of having the correct ingredients in the house can be a problem. Plan to have some staples that you keep on hand, so on the rare occasion when you forget a key ingredient or just could not make it to the store, you have enough to create a back up healthy meal. Keep a list on the pantry door to check off items you use or need to replace

In the Appendix there is a "Suggested Foods to Keep On Hand" list that will enable you to be prepared for changes in schedule or when meal fillers are needed.

Ideally, you enter the grocery store, list in hand, and stock the pantry and fridge with a weeks' worth of ingredients to feed your family the healthy meals you have so carefully planned. In reality, the time you have mentally blocked off to go to the store often gets re-assigned to other necessities: last minute school projects, working late without notice, pounding headaches, or a runaway dog that has to be found! How do we make it easier and more likely that the needed foods will be there when you get home to prepare dinner? Or better yet, someone else in the family makes dinner for you! Here are several ideas to make getting food in the house easier.

Online Shopping

Many major grocery stores have been offering this service for years. There is often a minor fee per order or a single fee for months or years worth of orders. If the fee feels expensive to you, remember, 1 or 2 impulse purchases made when hungry will cost more!

The wonderful benefits about the online shopping option are many:

Saved shopping lists

The foods you order can be saved and re-ordered in the future. So once you select the brand or size of a product you prefer, you just click to include it on future orders. You can even save different lists for re-use. For example, you can name a list "Cook-out" or "Week 1 menu," and if you choose to have the same menu again, just re-order the same list.

No Impulse Buying

This temptation is almost completely eliminated. Marketing professionals are masterful at positioning items that are on sale or special. These items are placed to attract your eye, especially at the end of aisles, and therefore increase the likelihood that you will put them in your cart and buy them. When ordering online, you are not victim to the marketing strategies or "specials."

Shopping When Hungry

This is another danger zone that is reduced or eliminated altogether. When you shop hungry, you tend to pick up what looks good right now and is placed at eye level – think candy in the checkout line! Even if you order online when hungry, you have a list and are not tempted as strongly by the sight of food, visually appealing packaging or the smell of fresh baked cookies!

Convenience

When ordering online, store hours are not an issue, so you do not have to block off a large period of time and the after work rush is not a factor. Ordering online also allows you to get dinner on the table faster. You can place your order while in your pajamas, during break time, or essentially any time you are able to do it. You are able to select the pickup time that best fits your schedule or better yet, send another family member to pick it up for you! If it is raining, snowing, cold or otherwise unpleasant weather, no problem. You pull up to the store, press the intercom button, they bring the bags out and put them into your car. You never even have to get out! The foods are even sorted by bag into frozen foods, refrigerated items, and dry grocery.

Grocery Delivery Services

This option sounds like something that went out of style years ago. But all good things come back, luckily!

It's not just the local, small town stores that offer this service either. Big name chain stores are in on this brilliant idea, so check with your local stores. There are also several online delivery services available that are not connected to a physical store. Amazon, under the name AmazonFresh, [fresh.amazon.com], Shipt, DirectEats, and Instacart are examples.

Delivery may have a fee or be a little more expensive than online shopping, or store pick-up, though it is another option and is very convenient. Most people actually save money because they eat at home more often. So by the time you save money by eating at home, avoid impulse buying and have healthier meals, the delivery fee is minimal.

A new option in my area is a service that sources local, organic foods as well as regular grocery items. They fill your order and deliver it to a specified pick up spot or to your house. There is no fee for pick up. They also deliver but there a fee for this option. You place the order online each week. Each day of the week there are multiple locations to choose from for pick up. TopGroceryDelivery.com lists them by city.

Seasonal Stock-Up

Local Farmers Markets are the best source when you want to stock up on fresh, local produce with a high nutrient value. When a food is shipped a great distance, the nutrient value drops each day. By purchasing local foods, and produce in particular, you are able to capture the highest nutrient value at the lowest price. When buying at the Farmers Market, you often get an even better price on larger quantities. Take what you cannot consume in a reasonable amount of time and freeze the rest. Check with your local Extension Service for the best methods of freezing for your locally grown foods.

Other sources are local farms, co-ops, produce delivery services and even road-side stands. The idea is to have high quality foods on hand to make meal preparation more likely.

Store Sales

Grocery and Big Box stores have foods on sale on a rotation. By knowing what you use often, and want to have on hand for quick, healthy meals, you can take advantage of these sales for healthy non-perishable staples.

Examples include whole grain pasta, brown rice, oatmeal, quinoa, dried beans & peas, whole grain cereals, canned tuna or salmon, nuts/seeds, dried fruit, etc. While saving money is a plus, having the basic ingredients on hand to prepare a quick healthy meal is the best reward.

Step Three: Prepare Ahead of Time

There is a menu planned. The food is in the house. Now it is time to quickly prepare the meal after a long day. This is where pre-prep comes in to help.

What is pre-prep? It is doing as much as possible ahead of time so the meal comes together quickly and easily. Pre-prep can include:

- Peeling, chopping, slicing or preparing produce
- Cooking meats ahead of time and refrigerating or freezing them
- Preparing casseroles to a specific point and cooking later

Having a selection of precut veggies and salad ingredients will increase how many servings of vegetables and salads your family eats in a week. Cutting and chopping produce a few days in advance will facilitate the preparation of a healthier meal. It can be like having a salad bar in your home – just open a few containers and build a delicious, colorful meal.

According to the USDA, cut or peeled produce loses a minimal amount of vitamins and nutrients after 5 -6 days. They lose about half their vitamin content in 1-2 weeks.

Meats are another food that benefits from pre-prep. Purchase a rotisserie chicken each week and use it for several meals. There are ideas for how to use one in the Recipe Section.

Roast your own. If you roast two or more chickens at once, you can dice the meat that you will not use this week and freeze for later use. See Recipe Section.

Marinate meats ahead of time. Place meat, chicken pieces, skirt steak, flank steak, pork chops, etc, in a zip top bag, add the marinade and close bag. You can now freeze the meat for later use but it will already be marinated. When you thaw it for cooking, it is ready and no additional marinating time is needed. Marinade ideas are in the Recipe section.

Other great time savers:
- Assemble ingredients in the pot or pan the night before. Then put the pan into the refrigerator until ready to cook. This works exceptionally well for crock-pot meals.
- Call home ahead of time and ask someone to pre-heat the oven or put a pot of water onto boil for faster meal prep.
- Pre-mix any dry ingredients for a recipe in a single container.
- Assemble casseroles or oven meals to the point of cooking and then freeze.

When my children were small and always hungry when we got home, I would use the pre-heat program on my oven. When we came home, the oven would already be at the desired temperature. I could take the pre-assembled pan out of the refrigerator and place directly into the hot oven. It saved at least 10 minutes, which is a lot of time when you have hungry toddlers – or adults! Not all ovens have this feature so check yours. If it does, try it out a few times when you are home to make sure it works correctly and safely.

Step Four: Cooking the Meal

The time has come – let the cooking begin! With proper planning, this part will go smoothly. The menu has been planned, the foods you need are in the house and preparing ahead has put you in a position to pull the meal together quickly.

One technique to streamline preparation is to use the same cooking method for all items. For example, all items might be cooked in the oven, on the grill, or in a skillet. An oven meal might include baked spaghetti, squash casserole and apple crisp. A grill meal could be grilled chicken, roasted corn on the cob and asparagus in a foil packet with Italian dressing.

If different cooking methods are being used, which to start first can be the key to having it all ready at once. This is a difficult thing to master and we all get better with time and experience. Anyone who has cooked Thanksgiving dinner knows what a challenge having all foods ready at once can be!

When planning the menu for the week, note how long items take to cook, according to the recipes or your experience. In general, the first thing to do when you arrive home is preheat the oven or grill, put water on to boil or heat the griddle.

Meats usually take the longest to cook, so plan to begin them as soon as possible. If a rice or pasta is on the menu, they need to be started as soon as the water is ready. Veggies steam quickly so can be the last item cooked.

Always work on another dish while waiting for the water to boil or oven to heat. You can chop all the veggies for the meal, get spices out of the cabinet, get pots and cooking utensils out, combine ingredients for another dish, even set the table or pack lunches for tomorrow. This way you have food out and can clean up everything at once.

For example, if the menu plan is for Baked Chicken, Wild Rice and Gingered Carrots, the timing could go this way.

Turn the oven on to preheat.
Put a pot of water on to boil.
Get the chicken out of the refrigerator, season and place in the baking dish. Place in the oven when heated. Bake according to recipe directions.
Get the rice out and measure the amount needed. Add to water when boiling. Follow package directions for cooking time.
Once chicken and rice are cooking, take carrots out of freezer or slice fresh carrots. Place them in a microwave safe dish with other ingredients, per recipe directions.

About 10 minutes before chicken and rice are done, begin to cook carrots.

If one item is ready before the others, you can place it in the oven to keep warm or on low heat.

Bonus Tips

In this section we will look at several ways to make meal prep easier, quicker and less stressful. The proper cookware, basic equipment, and short cuts are vital to successful meals.

Cookware

Suggested cookware is just that – suggested. It is not the final word. Cookware can be expensive and the price of a pot, pan or dish does not indicate how well it will work. I have had the same set of Revere Ware pots for over 25 years and use them daily. They have allowed me to feed my family well, and other than two cast iron skillets I bought because of want, not need, I have had no need for additional pans. Bargain shopper? You can pick up some great deals for cookware at Good Will, Consignment Shops, yard sales – often, they have never been out of the box!

Suggestions for cookware to have on hand include:

- Pyrex dishes in at least two sizes
- Sauce Pot in 1 qt, 2 qt, 3 quart
- Stock Pot or Dutch Oven
- Skillets with lids [cast iron are a good choice] 10" and 12"
- 1 deep skillet with 2" sides and a tight fitting lid. It might be called a Chef's Pan

- Griddle Pan – that covers 2 burners - this is great for pancakes or preparing multiple grilled cheese sandwiches or quesadillas at once
- Jelly Roll pans or cookie sheets, with a lip around edge
- Roasting Pan with rack

Basic Equipment

You can cook without some of the items listed here but these can make the job much easier. There are a lot of gadgets out there and I do not want you to fill your cabinets with items you will not use or clutter your counter tops. The goal is to have useful tools that do make meal prep easier and faster.

- Sharp Knives – Paring, Chef's 5-inch
- Cutting boards – one for meat, one for everything else
- Kitchen Shears [scissors]
- Box Grater
- Colander
- Microwave
- Rice cooker
- Crock Pot with removable dish
- Indoor Grill
- Blender - Immersion or regular
- Coffee Pot [for quick hot water]

- Vegetable Slicer/Mandolin
- Vegetable Chopper
- Salad Washer/Spinner

Short Cuts

Tips to make cooking faster and easier:

- Run water through a clean coffee maker then put into pot for quicker heating/boiling. Make sure to remove coffee grinds first!
- Crockpot meals – always double the recipe and use half for another meal.
- Eggs – hard-boil a half or full dozen during downtime and keep on hand for a quick breakfast, snack or to add to salads.
- Baked meats – bake double when possible and freeze or refrigerate leftovers.
- Place the most frequently used cookware items in one cabinet for easy access.
- Use leftover veggies to put in soups, stews, frittatas or omelets. You can freeze until you have enough to use.
- Pre-chop double the amount of veggies needed to use for another meal or salad.
- Prepare and place meats in marinade the night before they are on the menu.

- De-clutter your kitchen and stay organized. Set aside 15 minutes a day to clean out one cabinet, donate things you have not used in 1-2 years, replace cracked or broken items.
- Keep countertops clear so you can work quickly. Place used tools and utensils in the dishwasher or sink, especially if working with raw meat. This helps to avoid accidental cross contamination from raw meat to other foods, particularly uncooked foods.

Menu Planner

Use this menu planner weekly. Visit my website http://www.nutritionandrea.com/menu-planner-1/ to download the Excel spreadsheet. You can update it weekly and save for future use! [It is in color online!]

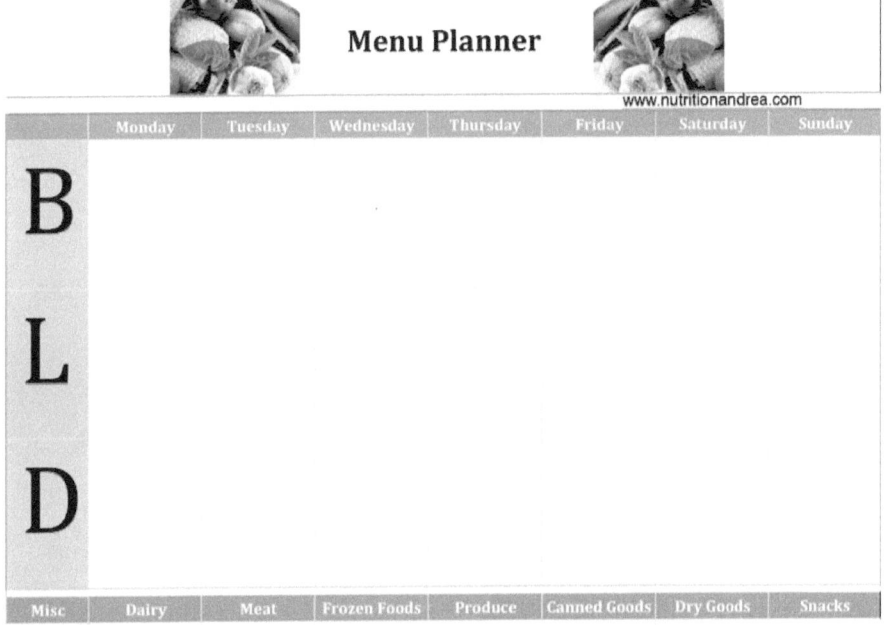

Mix and Match Meals

Select one item from each group to create a meal.

Protein
Baked Salmon/Fish
Skinless Chicken/Turkey Breast
Sirloin or Round Steak
Pork Loin Chop
1 Veggie/Bean Burger
2 TBSP Nut Butter
1 oz Nuts/Seeds
Tuna canned in water
2 eggs
¾ c cottage cheese, 2% fat
½ c beans
Ground meat in tomato sauce

Starchy Veggies/Grains
Brown Rice
Small Baked Potato
Mashed Potatoes
Corn
Whole Wheat Pasta
Butternut Squash
½ c beans
½ whole grain English muffin

2 inch square cornbread
6 whole grain crackers
2 slices low cal whole grain bread

Non-Starchy Veggies
Asparagus
Broccoli
Carrots
Tomato Slices
Spinach Salad
Brussels Sprouts
Yellow or Zucchini Squash
Tossed Salad
Cauliflower
Cucumber
Green Beans

Fruit
1 small apple
½ banana
15 grapes
½ c berries
½ c juice
½ c melon
¼ c dried fruit

Sample Menu Plans

*indicates recipe included

Slow Cooker Chicken Orzo and Garbanzo Beans*

Asparagus Frittata*

Teriyaki Chicken with Peanut Sauce*, Asian Slaw*

Chicken Picatta*, Feta Stuffed Tomatoes*, Whole Grain Angel Hair Pasta

Oregano Garlic Shrimp*, Brown Rice, Sliced Tomatoes

Pork Chops with Mustard Sauce*, Green Beans with Almonds*, Baked Sweet Potato

Cheesy Chicken, Broccoli and Rice Casserole, Fruit Yogurt Parfait*

Beefy Veggie Noodle Bake*, Baked Apple Slices*

Wash Day Beans*, Steamed Green Beans

Mexican Lasagna*, Mixed Green Salad

Rotisserie Chicken, Steamed Snow Peas, Wild Rice

Create Your Own Pizza*

Pasta with Jarred Pasta Sauce and Side Salad

Salad Bar Meal

Easy Crockpot Roast*, Baked Potato, Tossed Salad

White Chicken Chili*

Suggested Foods to Keep On Hand

Fresh Fruit and Vegetables

Baby Carrots

Celery

Apples

Pears

Grapes

Garlic – fresh

Onions

Riced cauliflower [maybe in the frozen section]

Meat and Alternate Proteins

Chicken, pork roast or tenderloin, ground meat

Beans – black, pinto, kidney, white, lentils. Dried or canned
[rinse before use]

Tofu or tempeh

Hummus

Eggs

Natural Peanut, Almond or other nut – butter

Raw nuts and seeds

Dairy

Plain organic yogurt

Sour cream

Cheese – variety of shredded: Mexican blend, cheddar, mozzarella, parmesan
Cheese – variety of block: 2%cheddar, pepper jack
Neufchatel-type cream cheese [reduced fat]

Frozen & Jarred/Canned Foods
Frozen meats – shrimp, salmon, chicken
Frozen vegetables – broccoli, spinach, carrots, mixed vegetables, soup blend, stir fry blend, others as desired
Frozen chopped or sliced onion and peppers
Frozen fruit - variety
Canned salmon, tuna, chicken
Canned or jarred tomato sauce, diced tomatoes
Salsa

Grains and Starches
Dried whole grain pasta
Whole Wheat couscous
Quinoa
Rice – brown or wild
100% Whole grain crackers

Recipes

Casseroles and Slow Cooker

Slow Cooker Chicken Orzo And Garbanzo Beans
Serves 6
Ingredients:
2 lbs Chicken breasts, boneless, skinless, cut into 12 cubes
1 can (16 oz) Garbanzo beans, reduced sodium, drained and rinsed
1 can (15 oz) Tomato sauce
1 1/2 cups Onion, diced
1/4 cup Olives, chopped
1 Tbsp Oregano, fresh, chopped
1 clove Garlic, minced
1/4 tsp Ground black pepper
12 oz dried orzo pasta, cooked
6 Tbsp Feta cheese, reduced fat, crumbled
Directions:
Add the chicken, beans, tomato sauce, onion, olives, oregano, garlic and pepper to the slow cooker and stir to combine.
Cover and cook on low until the chicken is cooked through, about 4 hours.
Cook the orzo pasta according to the directions on the package.

Serve over cooked orzo pasta and top each serving with a tablespoon of feta cheese. Garnish with a sprig of fresh oregano as desired.

Cheesy Chicken, Broccoli And Rice Casserole
Serves 6 -8
Ingredients
2cups cooked and chopped chicken
1 cup uncooked brown rice [measure 1 cup then cook]
2 cups broccoli [fresh or frozen]
¼ cup chopped onion
1/2 tsp garlic powder
 1 ½ tsp butter
½ cup Neufchatel cheese [light cream cheese]
1 1/3 cups milk
¼ tsp salt
1/8 tsp pepper
1/8 tsp ground nutmeg
½ cup grated Parmesan cheese
¼ cup shredded cheddar cheese [garnish]
1/3 cup fried onions [garnish]
Directions
Spray a 2-quart casserole dish with non-stick spray/olive oil.
Add the selected ingredients, through garlic powder.
Prepare sauce by melting butter in a 3-quart sauces pan, adding cream cheese and milk. Stir with a whisk until blended and smooth, about 2 minutes. Add salt, pepper and

nutmeg. Stir in Parmesan cheese with whisk and continue to stir for 3 minutes. Remove from heat.

Add to casserole and fold in to combine. The dish can be frozen at this point.
Sprinkle garnish on top. If frozen, allow to thaw in the refrigerator, then top with garnish.
Cover and bake at 350° for 45 – 50 minutes. Internal temperature should be 165°.

MICROWAVE DIRECTIONS
Combine as above, leaving garnish off. Cook at 50% power for 20 minutes. Stir.
Cook for an additional 10 minutes until internal temperature reaches 165°.
Top with garnish during last 5 minutes.

Beefy Noodle Bake
Serves 6 - 8
Ingredients
2 cups cooked ground beef, turkey or soy crumbles
2 cups uncooked whole wheat pasta [measure 2 cups dry then cook before adding to dish]
2 cups of mixed frozen vegetables
16 ounce can of diced tomatoes, undrained
½ cup chopped celery
¼ chopped onion
1 tsp chopped garlic

1 tsp dried salt free Italian Seasoning Blend

Garnish - 2 T Grated Parmesan cheese

Directions

Spray a 2-quart casserole dish with non-stick spray/olive oil.

Add the selected ingredients, except garnish, and stir to combine. The dish can be frozen at this point.

Sprinkle garnish on top. If frozen, allow to thaw in the refrigerator then top with garnish.

Cover and bake at 350* for 45 – 50 minutes. Internal temperature should be 165°.

Microwave Directions:

Combine as above, leaving garnish off. Cook at 50% power for 20 minutes. Stir.

Cook for an additional 10 minutes until internal temperature reaches 165°.

Mexican Lasagna

Serves 6

Ingredients

1 pound ground chicken breast

½ cup chopped onions

½ cup chopped peppers – green, red or yellow

2 ½ cups salsa

1 - 10 ounce box frozen corn

1 tsp garlic powder

1 tsp cumin

1 tsp chili powder

16 oz reduced-fat cottage cheese

12 corn tortillas

1 cup shredded reduced fat Mexican Blend cheese

Directions

Preheat oven to 375°.

Brown meat with onions and peppers.

Add seasonings, salsa and corn.

Layer lasagna in a 9"-by-12" pan that has been sprayed with olive oil.

Layer with 1/3meat mixture, and ½ tortillas& cottage filling.

Next, layer tortillas, cottage cheese.

Top with remaining meat sauce, then sprinkle with Mexican Blend cheese.

Cover with non-stick foil and bake for 30 minutes or until heated through.

Allow lasagna to stand for 5 minutes, then cut into cubes and serve hot.

Poultry, Beef, Pork & Fish

Teriyaki Chicken

Serves 4-6

Ingredients

4 Chicken breasts, skinless and boneless, cut into 1 inch cubes   [Or 1 block of firm Tofu, drained]

1 Tbsp olive oil

2 Tbsp low sodium teriyaki sauce

1 tsp lemon juice

Directions

Heat the olive oil in a skillet over medium heat.

Add cubed chicken.

Stir to sauté, for 3 minutes.

Add teriyaki sauce and lemon juice.

Continue to sauté, until chicken is cooked through, about 5 - 7 minutes.

Serve with Peanut Sauce.

Chicken Picatta

Serves 4

Ingredients

3 Tbsp flour

1 tsp paprika

½ tsp white pepper

¼ cup lemon juice

1 pound chicken breast [4 breasts]

2 Tbsp olive oil

½ white wine [or chicken broth]

2 Tbsp capers

Directions

Combine flour, paprika & white pepper in a shallow bowl.

Drizzle lemon juice over cutlets

Dredge breasts in flour mixture

Heat oil in a skillet over medium heat.

Sauté breasts for 2 minutes on each side, until browned.

Remove from skillet and keep warm

Add wine and 1 Tbsp lemon juice to skillet

Bring to boil while stirring

Add capers

Cook 1 minute

Pour caper sauce over breasts and serve.

White Chicken Chili

Serves 4

Ingredients

2 cans white beans, drained and rinsed

32 ounces chicken broth

1 tsp chili powder

1 tsp cumin

2 chicken breasts, cubed & cooked

1 small chopped onion

1 small can chopped chilies – not drained

Directions

1. Combine all ingredients in a large pot.

2. Heat over medium heat until bubbling.

3. Then reduce heat to low for one hour.

Easy Roast

Serves 6

Ingredients

Approx. 2 lbs lean eye of round roast (grain fed if possible and remove all fat)

32 ounces of beef stock

1 large onion, chopped

1 pound chopped carrots

3 cloves fresh garlic, chopped

Directions

Turn Crock-Pot on high.

Place roast in Crock-Pot.

Add 32 ounces of liquid beef stock

Chop onion, 3 cloves fresh garlic, and one pound of carrots; add to Crock-Pot as finished chopping.

After one hour turn Crock-Pot to low and cook for approximately 8 hours.

Insert meat thermometer to make sure roast has reached an internal temperature of 160 degrees.

Slice roast through and serve over couscous, quinoa, or noodles.

Pork Chops with Mustard Sauce

Serves 4

Ingredients

4 boneless, center cut pork chop

Salt

Pepper

1 TBSP mustard seed

1 TBSP olive oil

2 shallots, minced

1/3 cup dry white wine [or chicken broth]

1/3 cup half and half

2 TBSP Dijon mustard

2 tsp honey

Directions

Season pork chops with salt and pepper. Pat mustard seeds onto chops.

In a large skillet over medium high heat, heat the oil.

Add the pork chops and cook until pork is no longer pink, turning once. Time will vary based on thickness of chops. Sauté until golden brown.

Transfer onto a serving platter and keep warm.

Add shallots to pan. Reduce heat to medium and cook, stirring 1 minute.

Add the wine and broth and cook, stirring 1 additional minute.

Add the cream, mustard, and honey.

Stir until smooth and has small bubbles, about 1 minute.

Oregano Garlic Shrimp

Serves 4

Ingredients

1 pound shrimp, peeled and deveined

2 TBSP olive oil

1 TBSP garlic, minced

2 TBSP chopped fresh oregano

Salt, to taste

Pepper, to taste

Directions

In a bowl, combine shrimp, olive oil, garlic, oregano, salt and pepper. Mix well.

Heat skillet over medium heat. Add shrimp mixture and sauté for 3-4 minutes, or until the shrimp turn pink.

Salmon & Asparagus Packets

3 – 4 oz salmon

2 T chopped onion

1 tsp garlic powder

Salt/pepper

2 T low sodium soy sauce

¼ pound asparagus, trimmed

In a foil packet, combine all ingredients. Bake at 350° for 20 minutes or until fish flakes easily.

Ideas For Rotisserie Chicken

- Chicken Salad
- Chicken And Vegetable Soup
- Barbecue Chicken [Purchased BBQ Sauce]
- Chicken Topped Pizza
- In A Frittata
- Combine With Left Over Rice And Steamed Broccoli,
- Calzone Filling
- Sloppy Joe [Shred Chicken With Seasoning Mix],
- Chicken And Corn Chowder
- Stir Fry With Frozen Stir-Fry Vegetables.

VEGETARIAN

Asparagus Frittata
Serves 4
Ingredients
6 eggs
2 scallions, chopped
2 Tbsp olive oil
1/3 cup Parmesan cheese
24 asparagus spears, trimmed
1 tsp dried mint [optional]
Directions
Slice asparagus into 1-inch diagonal slices. Heat oil in a 10-inch non-stick skillet and sauté asparagus and scallions for 5 minutes.
Blend egg substitute, cheese, and mint. Pour over asparagus and scallions in skillet and cook on medium heat, gently pulling sides from skillet to cook eggs throughout.
Cover skillet with lid once egg mixture is cooked halfway through. Use a spatula to divide it into thirds. Turn each piece once. Serve immediately.

Wash Day Beans

Serves 6 – 8

Ingredients

2 cups black beans

1cup uncooked brown rice [measure 1 cup then cook before adding to dish]

16 ounces diced tomatoes, undrained

¼ chopped onion

¼ cup chopped olives

1 clove or 1 tsp chopped garlic

½ tsp cumin

Salt and pepper to taste

Garnish - ¼ cup shredded Mexican blend cheese

Directions

Spray a 2-quart casserole dish with non-stick spray/olive oil.

Add the selected ingredients, except garnish, and stir to combine. The dish can be frozen at this point.

Sprinkle garnish on top. If frozen, allow to thaw in the refrigerator then top with garnish.

Cover and bake at 350° for 45 – 50 minutes. Internal temperature should be 165°.

MICROWAVE DIRECTIONS

Combine as above, leaving garnish off. Cook at 50% power for 20 minutes. Stir.

Cook for an additional 10 minutes until internal temperature reaches 165°.

Pasta and Vegetables

Serves 4

Ingredients

1 Box Penne Pasta

2 Tbsp. Extra Virgin Olive Oil – (I love the infused Spice Infused Oils for this – it skips adding the spices!)

*Optional Ingredients (Chose your own)

1 bag steamed broccoli

1 jar drained artichoke hearts

2 cups washed spinach or 2 cups washed and chopped kale

1 can garbanzo beans, drained and rinsed or 1 can black beans, drained and rinsed

Directions

Cook Pasta, drain and rinse when done, according to box directions

Mix pasta with spinach or kale, steamed broccoli and beans. Toss mixture with Olive Oil.

Cauliflower Fried Rice

Serves 4

Ingredients:

2 cups cauliflower rice

2 tbsp coconut oil or olive oil, divided

3 large eggs, beaten

1/2 cup shredded carrots

2 tbsp finely chopped yellow onion

1/2 cup frozen peas

1/2 cup chopped mushrooms

1/4 cup reduced-sodium tamari

2 tbsp sesame oil

1/4 cup thinly sliced green onion

Salt, to taste

Instructions:

In a large sauté pan on medium-low, heat 1 tbsp coconut oil. Pour in whisked eggs, swirling them slightly to get a thin, even layer on the bottom of the pan. Continue to cook until just cooked through. Slide cooked eggs onto a cutting board and chop into a small dice. set aside.

Increase heat to medium-high and add remaining 1 tbsp coconut oil to the pan. Add carrots and sauté for 4 to 5 minutes. Add yellow onion, green peas and mushrooms. Sauté for 5 minutes.

Add cauliflower rice and cook for 5 – 8 minutes, stirring frequently until lightly browned and cooked through. Add tamari and mix well for 1 minute.

Turn off heat and add sesame oil, reserved cooked eggs. Mix well and season with salt. Top with sliced green onions.

SALAD IDEAS

Caesar - Romaine lettuce, kalamata olives, shaved parmesan cheese, croutons

Asian - Spinach, edamame, carrots, red cabbage, cucumber, crunchy lo mien noodles, sliced almonds

Mexicana - Romaine lettuce, black beans, cherry tomatoes, avocado, red onion, green pepper, corn, Mexican blend cheese

Greek - Romaine lettuce, quinoa, roasted red peppers, kalamata olives, cucumber, artichoke, feta cheese

Triple R - mixed lettuce, red onion, roasted red pepper, raisins, feta cheese, slivered almonds,

Cobb – mixed lettuce, chopped hardboiled egg, avocado, cherry tomatoes, red onion, bacon, blue cheese

Cheesy Apple– mixed lettuces, cucumber, diced apple, chickpeas, goat cheese, crunchy lo mien noodles,

Mediterranean – spinach, sun-dried tomatoes, kalamata olives, quinoa, red onion, toasted sesame seeds, feta cheese

Festive Fall – spinach, diced pear, red onion, dried cranberries, walnuts, blue cheese

Classic Spinach - Spinach, mushroom, red onion, chopped hardboiled egg, walnuts, goat cheese

Garden Party – spinach, cherry tomatoes, chopped broccoli, mushrooms, green peas, cucumbers, carrots, sunflower seeds

Colorful Crunch - Mixed lettuce, diced apple, feta cheese, cherry tomatoes, chopped broccoli, walnuts

Sunny Day - Romaine lettuce, edamame, raisins, sunflower seeds, carrots, cherry tomatoes

Add-Ins in addition to all above listed items
Grilled or baked chicken, baked or roasted turkey, tofu, tempeh, chopped kale, roasted corn, marinated beets, cauliflower, scallions, purple onions, broccoli slaw mix, banana peppers, grape/roma/vine tomatoes, reduced fat mozzarella cheese, parmesan cheese, kidney beans,

CREATE YOUR OWN PIZZA

This pizza is really yours to make! Add whatever toppings you would like. Mushrooms, green or red peppers and chopped red onions make great additions.
Serves 2-4

Ingredients
Crusts to choose from: Pre-prepared whole wheat pizza crust, whole grain English muffins or whole grain pitas
Extra Virgin Olive Oil
1 tsp. oregano
1tsp. minced garlic
1 tsp. basil
1 bag fresh spinach
1 whole tomato, sliced (optional)
¼ cup banana pepper (optional)
1 6 ounce bag shredded mozzarella cheese or 1.5 cups

Directions
Preheat oven to 400°.
Choose your crust.
Brush crust with extra virgin olive oil.
Evenly sprinkle basil, oregano and garlic over crust.
Place washed and patted dry spinach on crust. (it will seem like a lot, but it cooks down quickly)
Coat top with cheese.

Bake at 400° around 12 minutes until cheese is melted.
Remove pizza from oven.
Change oven to broil.
Add sliced tomato and banana peppers over cheese and broil about 3 minutes.
Let cool and slice and serve!

SIDE DISHES & SAUCES

Peanut Sauce

Serves 6

Ingredients

Makes about ½ cup or 4 servings

1 ½ Tablespoon smooth peanut butter

2 Tablespoons Canola Oil

2 Tablespoons reduced-sodium soy sauce

1 ½ Tablespoons sugar

2 teaspoons rice wine vinegar or white vinegar

½ teaspoon sesame oil

1/8 teaspoon cayenne pepper [ground red pepper]

Directions

Combine all ingredients in a small bowl and blend until well combined and smooth.

This sauce is good with chicken, tofu, or mixed grilled vegetables.

Control the level of spicy heat by adjusting the cayenne pepper. You can also add crushed red pepper to increase level of heat!

Cilantro Sauce
Makes: ½ cup
Ingredients
1 jar capers
1 cup cilantro
3 T olive oil
3 T green onions, chopped
Directions
Combine 2 T capers, 1 T caper brine, cilantro, olive oil, and 1 T water in the bowl of a small food processor. Process until smooth. Serve with grilled meat, as a salad dressing, over steamed vegetables, brown rice, quinoa, or whole grain couscous

Asian Broccoli Slaw
Serves 6 -8
Ingredients
1 bag of broccoli slaw
2 – 3 ounces sliced or slivered almonds. Can toast if desired. Can substitute peanuts [crushed] if desired.
1/4- 1/3 cup ginger salad dressing
Optional- ½ bag shredded carrots
Directions
Combine all and chill.

Feta Stuffed Tomatoes

Serves 8

Ingredients

4 large tomatoes

4 ounces Feta cheese, crumbled

¼ cup bread whole wheat crumbs

2 TBSP chopped scallions

2 TBSP fresh parsley, chopped

2 TBSP olive oil

¼ tsp salt

¼ tsp pepper

Directions

Pre-heat oven to 325°

Cut tomatoes in half horizontally. Scoop out pulp, leaving shells intact. Discard seeds and chop pulp.

Combine pulp, feta cheese and remaining ingredients.

Spoon mixture into shells and place in a 13 x 9 inch baking dish

Bake for 15 minutes.

Green Beans With Almonds

Serves 4

Ingredients

1 pound green beans

2 TBSP unsalted butter

2 tsp lemon juice

¼ cup unsalted almonds, toasted and chopped

¼ tsp kosher salt

Directions

Cook green beans in salted boiling water, for about 8 minutes or until crisp tender. Drain and place is serving bowl.

While green beans are cooking, add butter to a small skillet. Melt over medium heat and stir to prevent burning.

Add lemon juice, almonds and salt. Stir 30 seconds to toast almonds.

Toss gently with green beans.

Crispy Green Beans

Serves 1

Ingredients

¼ pound fresh green beans, washed and trimmed

2 TBSP olive oil

Directions

Toss green beans with olive oil. Place on baking sheet. Sprinkle with kosher salt, if desired. Bake at 425* for 15 minutes or until crisp.

Roasted Brussels Sprouts

Serves 4

Ingredients

1 pound fresh Brussels sprouts, washed and cut in half

Olive oil

Sale/pepper

Parmesan cheese (optional)

Directions

Toss Brussels sprouts in olive oil. Place on baking sheet. Sprinkle with salt and pepper. Roast at 375° for 10 minutes. Stir and roast for 5 – 10 minutes more. Check to make sure they do not burn. Remove from oven and sprinkle with Parmesan cheese, if desired.

Squash Casserole
Serves 4
Ingredients
1 lb yellow squash, diced
½ large onion, chopped
1 clove garlic, chopped
½ c mayonnaise
1 c 2% cheddar cheese, shredded, divided
1 egg
Seasoning blend
Directions
Steam squash, onion and garlic. Combine mayonnaise, ¾ cup cheese, and egg. Mix well.
In a greased baking dish, combine the squash mixture, mayonnaise mixture and seasoning blend. Top with the remaining ¼ cup of cheese. Bake at 350° for 40 minutes.

DESSERT

Fruit Yogurt Parfait
Serves 4
Ingredients
16 ounces Vanilla yogurt
1 cup fruit, can be mixed, berries, or single fruit
½ cup granola
Directions
In 4 dishes, layer yogurt and fruit. Repeat two times.
Top with 1 TBSP granola

Baked Apple Slices
Serves 4
Ingredients
4 medium Fuji or Granny Smith apples, sliced
1 TBSP cinnamon
1 tsp nutmeg
2 TBSP brown sugar
Water
Directions
Heat oven to 350°
Place sliced apples in a 9 x 9 baking dish,
Sprinkle with the combined cinnamon, nutmeg and brown
sugar.
Mix so that apples are coated.
Place 2 TBSP of water in the dish.
Bake uncovered 30 minutes

Pecan Date Bon Bons

Makes 8 -10

Ingredients

¾ c pecans

½ c pitted dates, chopped

2 tsp orange zest

Pinch sea salt

¼ tsp cinnamon

½ tsp white rice miso (up to 1 tsp per taste)

¼ c shredded unsweetened coconut

Directions

Preheat oven to 300°. Place pecans on a cookie sheet and roast for about 10 mins, until brown & toasted. Let cool. Put all ingredients except coconut in food processor. Pulse until you have an even texture. With moist hands, roll the mixture into 1-inch balls. Spread the coconut on a place and roll each ball in the coconut, covering each one evenly.

Chocolate Cottage Cheese Chia Pudding

Serves 1

Ingredients

1 c cottage cheese

1/3 c almond milk

1 heaping spoon cocoa powder

7 stevia drops

2 T chia seeds

Directions

Blend first four ingredients together. The desired consistency is milky, not too thick, so if you need more almond milk, add it in tablespoon by tablespoon until you achieve a milky consistency.

Add chia seeds and stir. Refrigerate overnight (or for a few hours if you're in a rush).

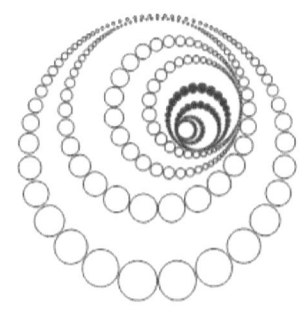

Nutrition Andrea

Andrea@NutritionAndrea.com
http://www.NutritionAndrea.com
Twitter @NutritionAndrea
Instagram Nutrition_Andrea
Facebook.com/NutritionAndrea

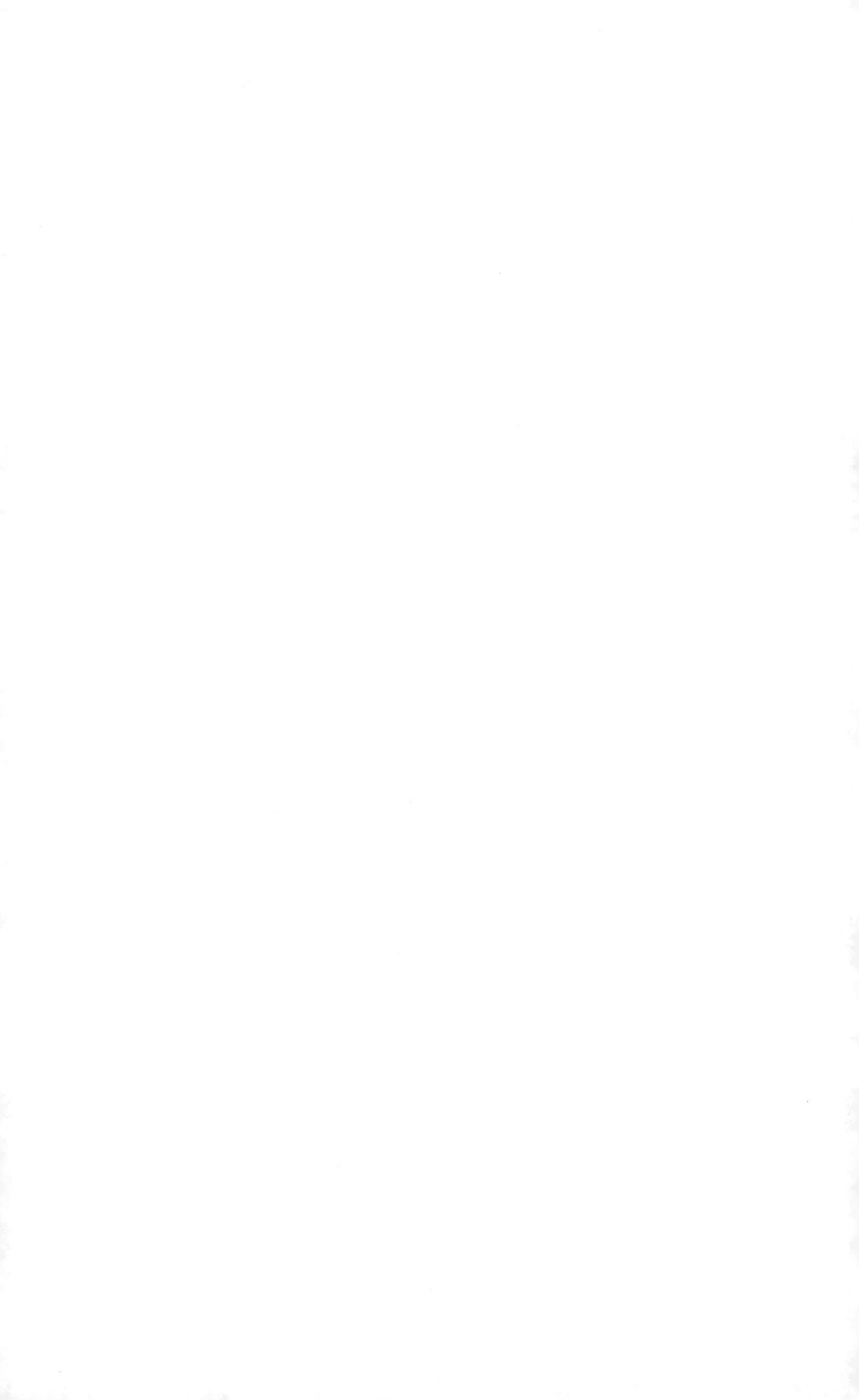

www.ingramcontent.com/pod-product-compliance
Lightning Source LLC
Chambersburg PA
CBHW020356290526
45785CB00005B/2304